INTERMITTENT FASTING FOR BEGINNERS

A Complete Guide To Intermittent Fasting: Boost Your Immunity, Reduce Inflammation, Accelerate Your Weight Loss. The Ultimate Guide To Overcome Ailments and Keep your Body and Spirit Healthy

PAUL BELFIORE

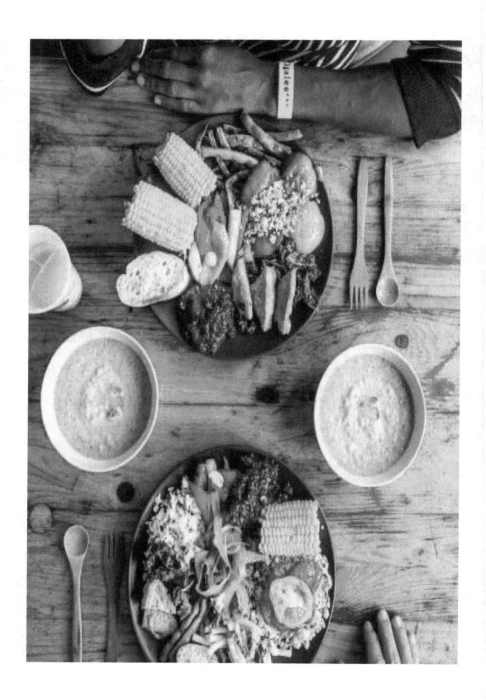

Table of Contents

INTRODUCTION

If you are tired of being too slow, too complicated, not always helpful, and what regimes cheer you on? Intermittent fasting can help you lose weight & gain health if you do it with common sense. We tell you everything. Intermittent fasting is not a diet but a new way of organizing the timing of food intake (meals) for maximum benefits. Individually, you don't change what you eat but when you eat it.

Intermittent fasting involves fasting for long hours (more than 12 hours), which is often like staying overnight and skipping breakfast, and then concentrating all of your meals for the day for a short period of time (for example, between 12 p.m. and 8 p.m.). It only refers to the food, but not to the drinks (don't be scared, you can have your coffee!).

Why does an intermittent diet seem like a good idea for anyone interested in losing weight but might want to know? Is intermittent intervention effective for the heart? There was another key aspect of intermittent fasting that can help you think about this to start a new trend. Intimate fasting is also known as almost always fine, but although some of these in them.

The American Journal of Clinical Nutrition conducted a relatively recent study that saw 16 men present and won a 10-week fight. In the next few days, the experts will consume approximately 25% of their previously estimated needs. The best has come out several queries, but he did not give us an oriented guide to follow. Unsurprisingly, the reasons for this experiment, at least, but what is still quite interesting was what she said. The gasps were pretty brilliant after just ten times, but have shown improvements in cholesterol, LDL chose, very helpful, and good pressure too. What made this an exciting discovery was the fact that most people had to lose more than these studies before seeing the same ideas. It was a fascinating discovery, which spurred a significant number of people to try.

RECIPES

1. Pan Chicken with Butternut Squash

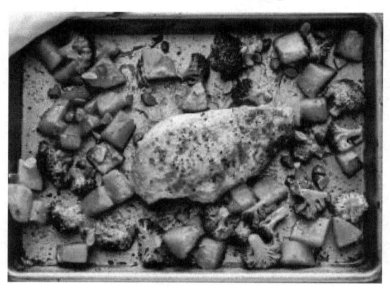

Prep Time: 15 Mins | Cooking Time: 20 Mins | Serve: 2

INGREDIENTS:

- 1 lb. of white ground chicken
- 1 lb. of tomatillos, chopped into a very large dice
- 1 small to medium butternut squash, peeled & cut into a small dice
- 2 small cans of diced green chiles
- 2 medium green chile peppers such as serranos

- 1 medium white onion, cut into a large dice
- 1 tablespoon coconut oil
- 2 teaspoon cayenne pepper
- 1 teaspoon paprika
- 1 teaspoon garlic powder

INSTRUCTIONS:

1. Put the coconut oil & spices in a pan on medium flame.
2. Put in the diced butternut squash along with the ground meat to the pan, occasionally turning until the meat is browned & squash is tender.
3. Put in the onion & chiles to the pan & mix. Remove the pan & put it aside. Layer the pan with the tomatillos & chiles
4. Pour the heated pan batter into the pan on top of the tomatillos—Cook for 4 hrs on low.

2.   Pan Coconut Mango Chipotle Chicken

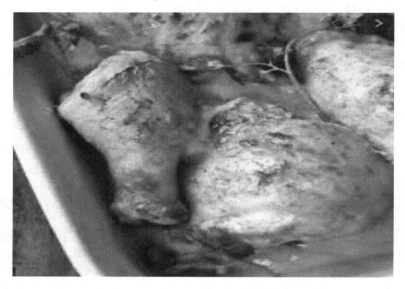

Prep Time: 15 Mins | Cooking Time: 25 Mins | Serve: 2

INGREDIENTS:

- 1 lb. of chicken breasts
- 1 can of coconut milk
- 1 large softball-sized mango, peeled & cubed
- 1 tablespoon of dried chipotle flakes

INSTRUCTIONS:

1. Pour the can of coconut milk into the cooking pan.

2. Put the mango cubes & the mango pit into the cooking pan.
3. Chop the chicken into cubes & put in it as well with the chipotle flakes & mix
4. well.
5. Cook for 5-6 hrs on low or for 3 hrs on high.

3.   Pan Chinese Chicken Thighs

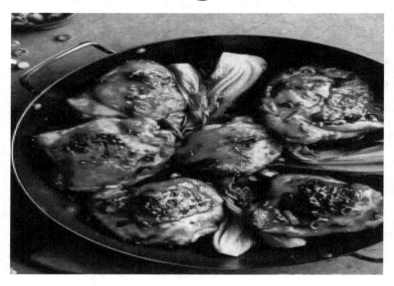

Prep Time: 20 Mins | Cooking Time: 25 Mins | Serve: 3

INGREDIENTS:

- 1.5 lbs. free-range pastured chicken thighs
- 1 large bunch of Collard Greens
- ½ mug hot Chinese mustard (should include only water, mustard seed, vinegar, & salt)
- 1 medium red onion, sliced
- Clove of garlic largely for every chicken thigh, sliced
- 2 teaspoon of ground cayenne pepper

- 1 teaspoon of red pepper flakes
- 1 tablespoon of coconut oil

INSTRUCTIONS:

1. Put the coconut oil in a heated pan & put the chicken thighs with sprinkles of cayenne pepper— Brown the chicken slightly.
2. Wilt the collard greens slightly in a microwave.
3. Combine the mustard with cayenne pepper, red pepper flakes & garlic in a casserole & stir well.
4. Grease the pan with coconut oil. Coat the chicken in the mustard batter & put each thigh in the center of a collard leaf
5. Top the chicken with a slice of onion & roll the leaf
6. Put some collards at the base of the cooking pan
7. Put the wraps on the collard green lining & cover the wraps on top with some collard leaves as well. Cook for 6 hrs on low.

4.   Pan Chicken Roll-Ups

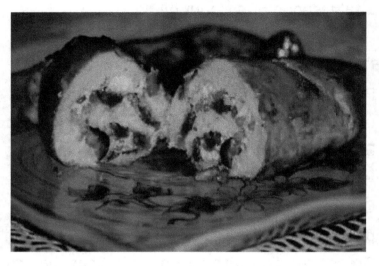

Prep Time: 10 Mins | Cooking Time: 20 Mins |
Serve: 2

INGREDIENTS:

- 4 boneless chicken breasts
- 6 to 8 slices of Prosciutto
- 1 bunch of asparagus Garlic cloves Salt & Pepper

INSTRUCTIONS:

1. Filet the chicken into halves & flatten with a meat mallet.
2. Trim the asparagus spears to the desired length.
3. Put the chopped garlic along with 3 strips of the asparagus inside the chicken

4. filet & roll-up.
5. Roll a slice of prosciutto around the chicken & poke a toothpick through to hold it together.
6. Put the rolls in the pan & cook for 4 hrs on low.

5.　Pan Curry Chicken with Peppers

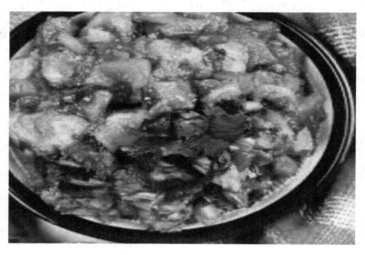

Prep Time: 15 Mins | Cooking Time: 30 Mins |
Serve: 2

INGREDIENTS:

- 1 to 1.5 lbs. of boneless chicken thighs, cut into cubes
- 1 or 2 cans of coconut milk
- 3 tablespoon Paleo-friendly Thai Kitchen Curry paste
- 1 small yellow onion
- 1 medium red bell pepper, cubes
- 1 medium green bell pepper, cubes
- ½ head of cabbage

INSTRUCTIONS:

1. Pour the coconut milk & the curry paste into the cooking pan.
2. Stir until the curry paste dissolves.
3. Put the chicken cubes & bell peppers in the pan & stir.
4. Chop the onions & put in into the chicken. Cut the cabbage into long strips & put it into the cooker & stir.
5. Cook covered for 4 hrs.

6. Pan Honey Garlic Chicken Wings

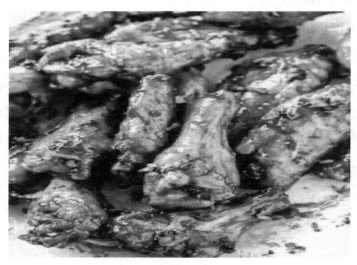

Prep Time: 15 Mins | Cooking Time: 25 Mins |
Serve: 3

INGREDIENTS:

- 2-3 lb. of wings
- ¾ mug of raw honey melted
- 1.5 tablespoons of minced garlic
- 2 tablespoons of olive oil
- ½ teaspoon sea salt
- ½ teaspoon pepper

INSTRUCTIONS:

1. Put the wings in the cooking pan. Combine the honey, garlic, olive oil, pepper & salt.

2. Pour the batter over the wings & stir so that the wings are covered.

3. Cut the cabbage into long strips & put it into the cooker & stir.

4. Cook for 3-4 hrs on high, or 6 hrs on low.

7. Pan Balsamic Chicken

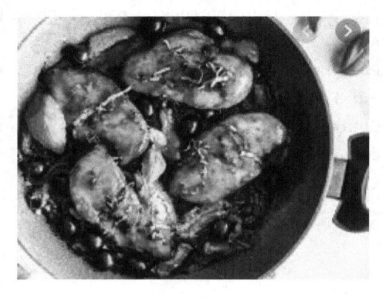

Prep Time: 15 Mins | Cooking Time: 20 Mins |
Serve: 2

INGREDIENTS:

- 4 boneless, skinless chicken breasts
- 6 fresh Italian sausage links
- 1 white onion, thinly sliced
- 4-6 cloves of garlic, chopped
- Extra virgin olive oil
- 2 teaspoon Italian seasoning
- 1 ½ teaspoon garlic powder
- 1 ½ teaspoon kosher salt
- 2 (14.5 oz.) cans organic diced tomatoes
- 1 (15 oz.) can tomato sauce

- 1 mug chicken stock
- ½ mug balsamic vinegar

INSTRUCTIONS:

1. Put the chicken breasts at the base of the pan & put a couple of tablespoons of olive oil.
2. Put in a teaspoon of Italian seasoning, a teaspoon of garlic powder & a teaspoon of Kosher salt. Put the sausages on top of the seasoned chicken.
3. Put a layer of onions & garlic & then put the diced tomatoes, tomato sauce, chicken stock & balsamic vinegar in the pot.
4. Sprinkle the remaining seasoning on top.
5. Cook for 5 hrs on low heat.

8. Pan Loaded Greek Chicken Breasts

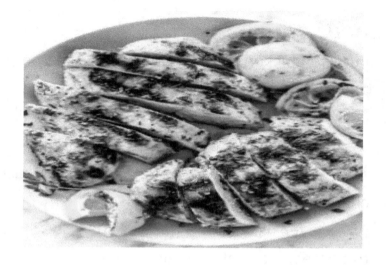

Prep Time: 10 Mins | Cooking Time: 25 Mins |
Serve: 2

INGREDIENTS:

- 4 – 6 boneless chicken breasts
- 1 Tablespoon olive oil
- ½ onion, diced
- ½ red pepper, cut into thin strips
- 2 pepperoncini peppers, cut into thin strips
- 6 oz. fresh spinach
- 2 teaspoon minced garlic
- 1 ½ teaspoon fresh oregano
- Salt & pepper Squeeze of lemon

- 1 mug chicken stock
- ½ mug white

INSTRUCTIONS:

1. Slit one side of each chicken breast to form a pocket.
2. Season the chicken with salt & pepper on each side.
3. Put some olive oil in a pan & sauté the onions & peppers for a few mins & put in in the spinach & garlic & cook until the spinach is wilted.
4. Sprinkle the oregano, salt & pepper. & remove from the flame.
5. Insert the spinach-pepper batter into the chicken pockets & put the chicken in the cooking pan.
6. Squeeze lemon juice over the chicken & put in the wine & chicken stock. Cook covered on low for 6-8 hrs or for 4 hrs on high.

9.   Mediterranean Pan Sour Chicken

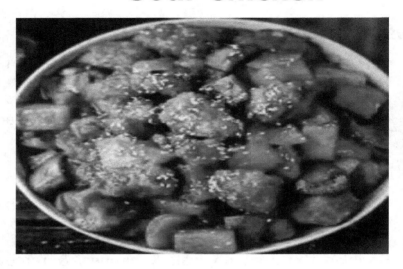

Prep Time: 20 Mins | Cooking Time: 25 Mins |
Serve: 3

INGREDIENTS:

- 1 small lemon (1 teaspoon of rind & 1 tablespoon of juice)
- 1 ¾ mug coarsely chopped onion
- ¼ mug pitted Kalamata olives, halved (12 olives)
- 2 Tablespoons drained capers
- 1 (14.5-oz.) can plum tomatoes, drained & coarsely chopped
- 12 bone-in chicken thighs (about 3 lbs.), skinned
- ¼ teaspoon freshly ground black pepper

- 1 Tablespoon olive oil
- Chopped fresh rosemary (optional)
- Chopped fresh parsley (optional)

INSTRUCTIONS:

1. Leave the lemon rind covered in a refrigerator.
2. Stir the onion, olives, tomatoes, capers with the lemon juice in a cooking pan.
3. Season the chicken thighs with pepper.
4. Pour oil into a heated pan & heat well.
5. Put half the quantity of the chicken in the pan & cook for about 2-3 mins per side.
6. Put the cooked chicken in the cooking pan.
7. Brown the rest of the chicken in the same way in the heated pan.
8. Cover with lid & cook for 4 hrs on low until the chicken is cooked.
9. Remove the chicken onto serving dishes.
10. Stir the refrigerated rind with the sauce & splash the sauce over the chicken.
11. Can be served garnished with rosemary or parsley.

10. Pan Chicken & Bacon

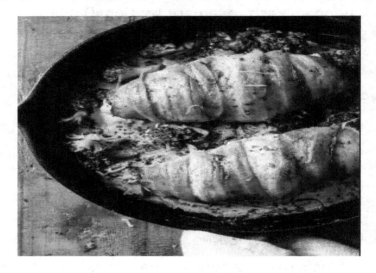

Prep Time: 15 Mins | Cooking Time: 30 Mins |

Serve: 2

INGREDIENTS:

- 5 chicken breasts
- 10 slices of bacon
- 2 tablespoon thyme (dried)
- 1 tablespoon oregano (dried)
- 1 tablespoon rosemary (dried)
- 2+3 tablespoon olive oil
- 1 tablespoon salt

INSTRUCTIONS:

1. Put all the ingredients in the pan & mix.

2. Cook for 8 hrs on low.

3. Shred the chicken & stir with 3 tablespoon

4. of olive oil.

11. Pan Coconut Chicken Drumsticks

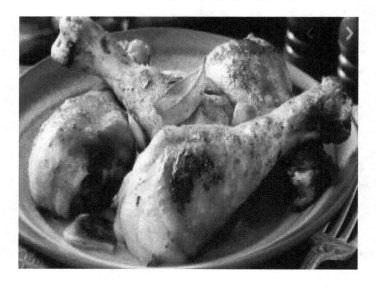

Prep Time: 15 Mins | Cooking Time: 20 Mins |

Serve: 2

INGREDIENTS:

- 10 drumsticks, skin removed
- 1 thick stalk fresh lemongrass, papery outer skins & rough bottom removed, trimmed to the bottom 5 inches
- 4 cloves garlic, minced
- thumb-size piece of ginger, sliced
- mug coconut milk
- Tablespoon Red Boat fish sauce
- Tablespoon coconut aminos

- 1 teaspoon five-spice powder
- 1 large onion, thinly sliced
- ¼ mug fresh cilantro, chopped Kosher salt
- Freshly ground black pepper

INSTRUCTIONS:

1. Season the chicken drumsticks with salt & pepper.
2. Blend the garlic, ginger, lemongrass, coconut milk, fish sauce, coconut aminos, spice powder in a blender until smooth.
3. Put the chicken with the sauce in the pan & cook on low for 6-8 hrs until the chicken is ready. Garnish with cilantro.

12. Pan Grilled Chicken & Peaches

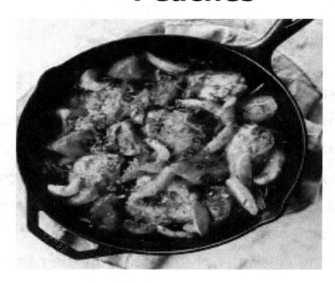

Prep Time: 15 Mins | Cooking Time: 25 Mins | Serve: 3

INGREDIENTS:

- 1 chicken
- 2-3 medium/large peaches, grilled
- 3 tablespoon coconut oil
- 1 tablespoon crushed red pepper
- ½ mug balsamic vinegar
- Sea salt & black pepper, to taste

INSTRUCTIONS:

1. Season the chicken with salt & pepper, including within the chicken cavity.

2. Put in a tablespoon of red pepper flakes with 2 tablespoon coconut oil & stir well, & apply it to the chicken.

3. Put the chicken in the pan & cook for 4-6 hrs on low.

4. Remove the chicken & put it aside. Put balsamic vinegar in a small pot & boil, reduce the flame & simmer until it thickens slightly; stir ring continuously. Shred the chicken.

5. Quarter the grilled peaches. Serve the chicken with the grilled peaches.

13. Pan Chicken with Sweet Potatoes

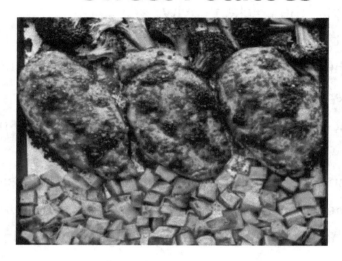

Prep Time: 15 Mins | Cooking Time: 20 Mins |
Serve: 2

INGREDIENTS:

- 2 sweet potatoes, peeled & cut into
- 1-inch chunks
- 1 lb. boneless, skinless chicken thighs Sea salt + cracked black pepper
- 2 cloves garlic, finely minced
- ½ mug chopped red onion
- 1 mug unsweetened apple sauce
- 2 teaspoon apple cider vinegar
- 1 tablespoon curry powder
- ½ teaspoon ground ginger Fresh basil, chopped

INSTRUCTIONS:

1. Layer the sweet potato chunks & the chicken at the bottom of the cooking pan. Put in salt & pepper.
2. Combine the garlic, red onion, apple sauce, cider vinegar, curry powder & ginger.
3. Put the batter over the chicken & sweet potatoes.
4. Cook covered for 6-8 hrs on low.
5. Garnish with basil.

14. Pan Green Chile Chicken

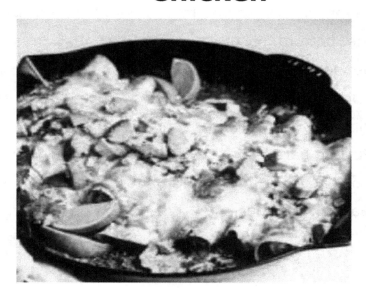

Prep Time: 20 Mins | Cooking Time: 30 Mins | Serve: 2

INGREDIENTS:

- 6 – 8 Boneless Skinless Chicken Thighs, thawed
- 1 (4 oz.) Can Green Chiles
- 2 teaspoon Garlic Salt
- ½ mug Diced Onions

INSTRUCTIONS:

1. Cook the chicken covered for 3 hrs in a pan on high.

2. Drain the juices from the cooking pan. Combine the green chiles, garlic salt & onions & pour over the chicken & cook covered for another 30 mins

3. more on high.

4. Shred the chicken & spoon some batter wrapped up in burritos & serve.

15. Pan Creamy Mexican Chicken

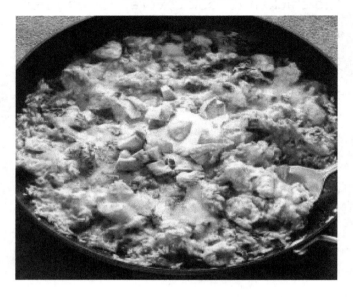

Prep Time: 10 Mins | Cooking Time: 25 Mins |
Serve: 2

INGREDIENTS:

- 1 mug sour cream
- ½ mug chicken stock 1 - 14 oz. can diced tomatoes & green chilies
- 1 batch homemade taco seasoning
- 2 lbs. chicken breast

INSTRUCTIONS:

1. Put in the chicken stock, sour cream, diced tomatoes with green chilies & taco seasoning to the pan & stir well.
2. Put in the chicken breasts to the crockpot.
3. Cook covered for 6 hrs on low.

16. Pan Buffalo Chicken Lettuce Wraps

Prep Time: 15 Mins | Cooking Time: 20 Mins |
Serve: 3

INGREDIENTS:

For the chicken:

- 24 oz. boneless skinless chicken breast
- 1 celery stalk
- ½ onion, diced
- 1 clove garlic
- 16 oz. fat-free low sodium chicken broth
- ½ mug hot cayenne pepper sauce
- For the wraps:
- 6 large lettuce leaves, Bibb
- 1 ½ mugs shredded carrots
- 2 large celery stalks, cut into 2-inch matchsticks

INSTRUCTIONS:

1. Put the chicken, celery stalks, garlic & broth in a pan & cook covered on high for 4 hrs.
2. Remove the chicken & shred it. Retain only half a mug of broth in the pan & throw out the rest.

3. Put the shredded chicken back to the pan with the hot pepper sauce & cook for an extra 30 mins on high. For the wraps, put half a mug of buffalo chicken on each lettuce leaf with

4. ¼ mug carrots, celery & your favorite dressing & wrap.

17. Pan Pesto Salad

Prep Time: 15 Mins | Cooking Time: 25 Mins |
Serve: 2

INGREDIENTS:

- 1.5 lb. organic boneless chicken breasts (3 or 4 pieces)
- 1 garlic clove, chopped ½ white onion, chopped
- 1 mug organic chicken broth
- ¼ teaspoon garlic powder
- Dash of salt & freshly ground pepper
- Pesto Sauce:
- 1 mug fresh basil
- 1 ½ mug spinach
- ½ mug cashews, walnuts, or nuts of choice
- 1 tablespoon extra-virgin olive oil
- 1 garlic clove
- ½ lemon, juiced
- Dash Himalayan sea salt to taste
- Dash Freshly ground pepper to taste
- Dash red pepper flakes
- ¼ mug pine nuts

INSTRUCTIONS:

1. Put the chicken breasts along with the broth in the pan & put in garlic, onion, garlic powder, salt & pepper to it.

2. Cook on high for 3 hrs & then remove the chicken & shred it. For the pesto sauce, combine all the sauce ingredients other than the oil in a food processor & pulse it until it is ground. Put in the oil & pulse again. Combine the chicken & the sauce in a casserole.

3. Toast the pine nuts for around 3 mins in a pan.

4. Top the salad with pine nuts & refrigerate for some time.

18. Pan Sweet Garlic Chicken

Prep Time: 10 Mins | Cooking Time: 20 Mins |
Serve: 2

INGREDIENTS:

- 4 chicken breasts
- ¼ mug raw honey
- ¼ mug apple cider vinegar
- 2 tablespoons fresh lemon juice
- ¼ mug chicken stock
- 3 tablespoon garlic, minced
- 2 tablespoon coconut aminos
- 2 teaspoon tapioca starch
- 2 tablespoon water
- Red pepper flakes, to taste
- Sea salt & freshly ground black pepper

INSTRUCTIONS:

1. Stir the honey, vinegar, lemon juice, coconut aminos, garlic, salt, pepper & chicken stock in a casserole.
2. Put the chicken in the pan & pour the sauce over it.

3. Cook covered for 6-8 hrs on low. Remove the chicken & put it aside. Pour the sauce into a saucepan & heat. Stir the water with the tapioca starch until dissolved & put into the sauce.

4. Stir the sauce until it thickens. Sprinkle red pepper flakes on the chicken & pour the sauce over it.

19. Pan Chicken Tikka Masala

Prep Time: 20 Mins | Cooking Time: 25 Mins |
Serve: 2

INGREDIENTS:

- 2 tablespoon olive oil
- 6 chicken thighs boneless, skinless, cut into 1" pieces
- 1 yellow onion diced
- 2 teaspoon garlic minced
- 2 teaspoon coarse salt
- 1 ½ tablespoon garam masala
- ½ teaspoon paprika
- 3 tablespoon tomato paste
- 28 oz. canned diced tomatoes
- 15 oz. coconut milk
- Cilantro to garnish

INSTRUCTIONS:

1. Brown the chicken breasts in oil in a pan & then transfer it to the cooking pan. Sauté onion in the pan & then put in garlic, salt, paprika & garam masala & sauté.

2. Put the tomato paste in the pan & cook for a min; after which, put in the tomatoes & simmer.
3. Pour the entire tomato sauce & the coconut milk into the pan over the chicken.
4. Cook covered for 4 hrs on high or 6-8 hrs on low.
5. During the last 30 mins of cooking, uncover the cooker & allow the sauce to thicken slightly.
6. Garnish with cilantro.

20. Pan Cashew Chicken

*Prep Time: 15 Mins | Cooking Time: 25 Mins |
Serve: 3*

INGREDIENTS:

- ¼ mug arrowroot starch
- ½ teaspoon black pepper
- 2 lbs. chicken thighs, cut into bite-size pieces
- 1 tablespoon coconut oil
- 3 tablespoon coconut aminos
- 2 tablespoon rice wine vinegar
- 2 Tablespoon organic ketchup
- ½-1 tablespoon palm sugar
- 2 minced garlic cloves
- ½ teaspoon minced fresh ginger
- ¼-1/2 red pepper flakes
- ½ mug raw cashews

INSTRUCTIONS:

1. Put the chicken, starch & black pepper in a Ziploc bag & seal it. Toss t coat the chicken.

2. Put coconut oil in the heated pan & put in the chicken to it & brown on both sides. Transfer the chicken to the cooking pan. Combine the coconut aminos with the red pepper flakes in a casserole & pour it over the chicken & stir.

3. Cook covered for 3-4 hrs on low. Put in the cashews & stir in the sauce prior to serving.

21. Pan Almond Butter Chicken

Prep Time: 15 Mins | Cooking Time: 20 Mins |
Serve: 2

INGREDIENTS:

- 1-2 lbs. chicken breasts
- ½ mug almond butter
- 2 teaspoon cumin
- 1 teaspoon crushed garlic
- 1 lime, juiced
- ¼ mug GF soy sauce
- ½ mug chicken broth

INSTRUCTIONS:

1. Grease the pan with a cooking spray & put the chicken to the bottom.
2. Put in the cumin, garlic & almond butter.
3. Put in the soy sauce, chicken broth & squeeze lime over the chicken & stir well.
4. Cook covered for 4 hrs on high or 6-8 hrs on low flame.

22. Pan Chicken Masala

Prep Time: 15 Mins | Cooking Time: 25 Mins |
Serve: 2

INGREDIENTS:

- 5 boneless, skinless chicken breast halves, cut into 1-inch pieces (about 32oz)
- ½ large yellow onion, finely diced
- 4 cloves garlic, minced
- 2 tablespoon fresh, finely grated ginger
- 3 oz. tomato puree
- 1 mug cashew crème
- 1 ½ mug almond milk
- 2 tablespoon extra virgin olive oil
- 2 tablespoon lemon juice
- 2 tablespoon garam masala
- 1 tablespoon ground cumin
- ½ tablespoon paprika powder
- 2 teaspoon Celtic sea salt, or to taste
- ¾ teaspoon cinnamon powder
- ¾ teaspoon freshly ground black pepper
- 1-3 teaspoon cayenne pepper
- 1 red pepper, sliced in half & seeds removed
- 2 bay leaves

- 1 tablespoon arrowroot powder
- Chopped cilantro for serving

INSTRUCTIONS:

1. To make the sauce, combine chopped onions, minced garlic, tomato puree, grated ginger, cashew crème, ½ mug almond milk, olive oil, garam masala, lemon juice, cumin, paprika, salt, cinnamon, pepper & cayenne pepper & stir well.
2. Put the chicken in the cooking pan, and
3. pour over the sauce & stir to ensure the chicken is coated with the sauce.
4. Put in the bay leaves & the red pepper.
5. Cook covered for 6 hrs on low. 30 mins before completion of cooking, whisk a mug of almond milk & arrowroot & pour the batter into the pan & stir.
6. Prior to serving, remove the bay leaves & red pepper & top the chicken with cilantro.

23. Pan Honey Mustard Chicken II

Prep Time: 10 Mins | Cooking Time: 30 Mins |
Serve: 2

INGREDIENTS:

- 6 chicken breasts
- ¼ mug honey
- ½ mug Dijon mustard
- ½ mug chicken broth
- 1 tablespoon hemp hearts

INSTRUCTIONS:

1. Whisk the mustard, honey & broth together & coat the chicken with the batter.
2. Put the chicken breasts in the pan & pour the remaining honey-mustard batter over the chicken.
3. Cook for 3 hrs on high & for another 3 hrs on low.

24.   Pan Hot & Spicy Chicken

Prep Time: 20 Mins | Cooking Time: 20 Mins |
Serve: 2

INGREDIENTS:

- 2 sweet onions, sliced
- 1 teaspoon sea salt
- 2 teaspoon paprika
- 1 teaspoon garlic powder
- 1 teaspoon poultry seasoning
- ¼ teaspoon cayenne pepper
- ¼ teaspoon chipotle chili powder
- ½ teaspoon freshly ground black pepper
- 1 (5 to 6-lb.) organic chicken, rinsed & patted dry

INSTRUCTIONS:

1. Put the onion slices at the bottom of
2. the cooking pan.
3. Stir all the spices in a casserole & rub it on the chicken.
4. Put the chicken on the onions & cook covered for 5-6 hrs on low.

25. Pan Moroccan Chicken

Prep Time: 15 Mins | Cooking Time: 25 Mins |
Serve: 3

INGREDIENTS:

- 1 (14 oz.) can of Tomato Sauce
- ⅓ mug of Apricot Puree Juice of
- 1 small Lemon
- 1 teaspoon of Cumin
- 1 teaspoon of ground Ginger
- 1 teaspoon of Salt
- ½ teaspoon of Sweet Paprika
- 4 lbs. of Chicken Thighs
- 2 Yellow Onions, sliced
- 3 Garlic Cloves, minced
- 1 Tablespoon of Fresh Grated Ginger
- 3 Cinnamon Sticks
- ⅓ mug of Almond Butter
- 1-2 mugs of Water
- 3 tablespoon of coconut oil

INSTRUCTIONS:

1. Stir the tomato sauce, lemon juice, apricot, cumin, ground ginger, salt & paprika in a casserole.
2. Fry the chicken on both sides in a pan with coconut oil & then transfer the chicken into the cooking pan.
3. Put onions, garlic & ginger into the pan & sauté & then transfer to the cooking pan.
4. Remove the pan from the flame & put in the sauce batter to the pan & stir a mug of water & almond butter in it. Pour it into the pan & put in cinnamon sticks.
5. Put in water if required to slightly cover
6. the meat & cook covered for 6 hrs on low.

26. Pan Orange Chicken

Prep Time: 15 Mins | Cooking Time: 25 Mins |
Serve: 2

INGREDIENTS:

- 2 chicken breasts, cut into 1-inch cubes
- 1 Onion, diced
- 1 tablespoon grated ginger
- 1 large orange, zest & juice squeezed out, about
- ¼ mug of juice
- 3 Cloves crushed & sliced garlic
- ¼ mug Chicken stock
- 1 teaspoon chili flakes
- ½ teaspoon apple cider vinegar
- 3 tablespoon honey or maple syrup
- ½ teaspoon paprika
- 2 teaspoon Sesame Oil
- 1 tablespoon sesame seeds

INSTRUCTIONS:

1. Put the chicken breast pieces in a cooking pan.
2. Stir all the ingredients other than the sesame oil & seeds & pour over the chicken.

3. Toss the chicken into the batter. Cook on high for 2-3 hrs or for 4-6 hrs on low.

4. Stir in the sesame oil & seeds once ready.

27. Pan Walnut Chicken

Prep Time: 10 Mins | Cooking Time: 20 Mins |
Serve: 2

INGREDIENTS:

- 2 mugs toasted walnuts
- 3 tablespoon olive oil, divided
- 2 onions, chopped
- 1/3 mug pomegranate molasses
- ½ mug chicken stock 2 tablespoon lemon juice
- 1 ½ teaspoon cinnamon
- 1 teaspoon turmeric
- 2 tablespoon brown sugar
- 1 teaspoon kosher salt
- ½ teaspoon ground pepper
- 8 bone-in, skin-on chicken thighs
- 10 peeled garlic cloves 4 stems of fresh rosemary
- 4 carrots, chopped into 1" pieces
- 1 mug pomegranate seeds
- ½ mug chopped parsley

INSTRUCTIONS:

1. Blitz the toasted walnuts in a food processor until coarse.

2. Sauté onions in a pan of olive oil & put in the toasted walnuts & cook for another 2 mins.

3. Put in the pomegranate molasses, chicken stock & lemon juice & stir well & pour into a casserole.

4. Combine turmeric, cinnamon, brown sugar, salt & pepper & coat each piece of the chicken with the spices. Brown the chicken on both sides with some olive oil in the pan.

5. Put the chicken in a pan & put the onions & walnut gravy over it. Throw in the garlic cloves & the rosemary stems.

6. Until the gravy begins to bubble, the pan should be on a high; after that, reduce to low & cook for 3 hrs.

7. Put in the carrots & cook for another 1 ½ hr.

8. Garnish topped with parsley & pomegranate seeds.

28. Pan Curry Coconut Chicken

Prep Time: 20 Mins | Cooking Time: 25 Mins |
Serve: 2

INGREDIENTS:

- 1 to 1.5 lbs. of boneless chicken breast, diced
- 2 cans of coconut milk
- 3 Tablespoon red curry paste
- 1 small yellow onion, diced
- ½ medium red bell pepper, chopped
- ½ medium green bell pepper, chopped
- ¼ head of cauliflower, chopped
- ¼ head of cabbage, chopped
- 3 cloves of garlic, minced

INSTRUCTIONS:

1. Put the chicken broth & the coconut
2. milk into the pan set on low. Put in the curry paste & stir until it dissolves.
3. Put in the chicken, onions & bell peppers & stir.
4. Put in the cauliflower florets, cabbage & garlic to the cooking pan. Cook covered for 4 hrs.

29. Pan Okra Chicken

Prep Time: 15 Mins | Cooking Time: 30 Mins |
Serve: 2

INGREDIENTS:

- 4 bone-in chicken legs
- ¾ teaspoon kosher salt, divided
- ½ teaspoon freshly ground pepper, divided
- 3 teaspoon canola oil, preferably organic, divided
- 4 cloves garlic, finely chopped
- 2 large onions, sliced
- 1 ½ teaspoon dry Italian seasoning
- ½ mug dry red wine
- 1 28-oz. can diced tomatoes
- 1/3 mug chopped green olives
- 2 bell peppers any color, or 4 cubanelle peppers, cored & sliced
- 3 mugs fresh or frozen sliced okra
- ½ mug chopped flat-leaf parsley

INSTRUCTIONS:

1. Season the chicken pieces with salt & pepper.

2. Brown the chicken in a heated pan with olive oil over medium flame & transfer the chicken to the insert of the cooking pan.

3. Sauté the garlic, onions, Italian seasoning, some salt & pepper for around 2 mins & pour into the cooking pan.

4. Pour the wine into the heated pan & bring to a simmer continuously stir ring.

5. Put in the tomato & olives & bring to simmer on high flame & transfer to the cooking pan.

6. Put the peppers in the pan & cook on low for 8 hrs.

7. Just prior to the last 30 mins of cooking, layer the okra on top & cook covered for the next 30 mins.

30. Pan Chicken Teriyaki

Prep Time: 15 Mins | Cooking Time: 20 Mins |
Serve: 3

INGREDIENTS:

- 2 lbs. chicken breast or thighs, boneless & skinless
- ¾ mug soy sauce
- ⅓ mug sugar
- ¼ mug water
- 1-inch fresh ginger, grated
- 4 green onions, chopped
- 2 tablespoon sesame seeds

INSTRUCTIONS:

1. Put the chicken in the cooking pan. Combine the sugar, soy sauce, water & ginger in a casserole & pour it over the chicken.
2. Cook covered on low for 5-6 hrs or for 2-3 hrs on high.
3. Once ready, slice the chicken & garnish with sesame seeds & green onions.

31. Pan Chinese Spiced Chicken

Prep Time: 10 Mins | Cooking Time: 25 Mins |

Serve: 2

INGREDIENTS:

- 1 stalk celery- cut into 1-inch pieces
- 3 green onions - sliced into 1-inch pieces
- 4 to 5 lb. roasting chicken
- 1 Tablespoon soy sauce
- 2 teaspoon Chinese 5 spice powder

INSTRUCTIONS:

1. Put the onion & the celery inside the chicken cavity.
2. Combine the soy sauce & the spice & rub over the chicken.
3. Transfer the chicken to a pan & cook for 6-7 hrs on low.
4. Put the chicken in a broiler-safe pan for 5 mins under the oven broiler. Throw out the veggies & serve.

32. Pan Maple Cranberry Apple Chicken

Prep Time: 15 Mins | Cooking Time: 25 Mins |
Serve: 2

INGREDIENTS:

- 1 lb. chicken thighs, boneless & skinless
- 1 medium white onion, sliced
- 2 medium sweet potatoes, peeled & diced
- 2 medium apples, peeled & diced
- ¾ mug fresh cranberries
- 2 tablespoon olive oil
- 3 teaspoon maple syrup
- 1 teaspoon pumpkin pie spice
- Extra dash nutmeg
- Dash of salt
- Dash of pepper

INSTRUCTIONS:

1. Put some olive oil into the cooking pan. Put the chicken in the pan & put in the maple syrup & spices to it.

2. Put in the sweet potatoes, apples, onion & cranberries to the cooking pan. Cook for 4-5 hrs on low.

3. Stir well using a spoon & then cook again for around 30 mins.

33. Pan Almond Chicken Thighs

Prep Time: 20 Mins | Cooking Time: 20 Mins |
Serve: 2

INGREDIENTS:

- 1 tablespoon olive oil
- 8-12 large olives stuffed with pimentos
- ½ mug raw almonds
- 1 cloves garlic, minced
- ¼ onion, coarsely chopped
- ¼ teaspoon black pepper
- ½ teaspoon cumin
- ½ teaspoon chili powder
- ½ mugs chicken broth
- 4 boneless, skinless chicken thighs

INSTRUCTIONS:

1. Grease the pan with olive oil. Stir all the other ingredients other than the chicken in the cooking pan.
2. Put the chicken in & toss it in the batter.
3. Cook for 8 hrs on low until the chicken is done.

34. Pan Thai Chicken

Prep Time: 15 Mins | Cooking Time: 25 Mins |
Serve: 2

INGREDIENTS:

- 1 ½ tablespoon green curry paste
- ¼ mug chicken broth
- 1 14 oz. can coconut milk
- 3 tablespoon fish sauce
- 2 tablespoon agave nectar
- 2 lbs. chicken, chopped into bite-sized pieces small onion, chopped
- 1/3 mug carrot matchsticks
- 1 mug mushrooms, chopped
- 2 mugs cauliflower florets, chopped

INSTRUCTIONS:

1. Stir the first five ingredients in the pan & mix.
2. Put in all the remaining ingredients & stir well to combine.
3. Cook for 6-7 hrs on low.

35. Pan Indian Curry Chicken

Prep Time: 10 Mins | Cooking Time: 30 Mins | Serve: 3

INGREDIENTS:

- 1.5 lbs. boneless, skinless chicken thighs
- 1 (13.5 oz.) can coconut milk
- 1 tablespoon agave nectar
- 1 tablespoon red chili paste
- 1 tablespoon curry powder
- 1 teaspoon fish sauce
- 3-4 cloves garlic, diced
- 1-inch knob of ginger, diced
- 1 onion, sliced
- 1 green pepper, diced
- 2-3 sweet potatoes, diced

INSTRUCTIONS:

1. Combine the coconut milk, curry powder, fish sauce, ginger, agave & red chili paste in a cooking pan.
2. Put in the chicken & toss it in the sauce.
3. Put in the veggies on top.

4. Cook for 7-8 hrs on low.

36. Pan Stuffed Chicken Breast

Prep Time: 10 Mins | Cooking Time: 25 Mins |
Serve: 2

INGREDIENTS:

- 2 plump chicken breasts, thawed
- 1 mug shredded carrots
- 1 mug shredded zucchini
- 2 cloves garlic, finely minced
- 1 tablespoon lemon juice
- 1 tablespoon olive oil
- 1 teaspoon crumbled dried sage

INSTRUCTIONS:

1. For the stuffing, stir all the ingredients other than the chicken in a casserole

2. Cut the chicken breasts up to the middle to make a pocket.

3. Scoop the stuffing into the chicken pockets & secure the ends with toothpicks.

4. Put the chicken in the pan cook for 4 hrs on low until the chicken is ready.

37. Pan Honey Sesame Chicken

Prep Time: 15 Mins | Cooking Time: 20 Mins |
Serve: 2

INGREDIENTS:

Chicken:

- 3 lbs. boneless, skinless chicken thighs or breasts
- Sea salt - to taste
- Freshly ground black pepper - to taste
- 1 yellow onion, small, peeled & roughly chopped
- 3 garlic cloves ½ mug raw honey
- 1/3 mug Paleo ketchup ½ mug coconut aminos
- 2 Tablespoon toasted sesame oil
- ¼ teaspoon crushed red pepper
- 1 Tablespoon arrowroot powder (optional)

Veggies:

- 1 bunch rainbow chard, cut lengthwise into one-inch ribbons
- 2 mugs broccoli, cut into bite-sized pieces
- 1 red bell pepper, cored & thinly sliced lengthwise
- 1 Tablespoon coconut oil
- 1 teaspoon coconut aminos
- ½ teaspoon toasted sesame oil Sea salt - to taste
- Freshly ground black pepper - to taste

Garnish:

- 1 teaspoon sesame seeds
- 3-4 green onions, thinly sliced

INSTRUCTIONS:

1. Season the chicken with salt & pepper and put in a cooking pan.
2. Put all the other chicken ingredients except the arrowroot powder in the food processor & pulse until the liquid ingredients are well combined.
3. Pour the batter over the chicken in the pan & cook for 3 hrs on low. Remove & shred the chicken.
4. Whisk the arrowroot powder in the broth that's left in the pan & cook for 5 mins.
5. Put in the chicken back to it & mix. For the veggies, put coconut oil in a heated pan & sauté the veggies till the bell pepper & broccoli are tender & the chard is wilted. Put in the remaining ingredients & mix.
6. Put the veggies in a serving tray & put the chicken batter on top of it. Garnish with sesame seeds & green onion.

38. Pan Balsamic Chicken

Prep Time: 15 Mins | Cooking Time: 25 Mins |
Serve: 2

INGREDIENTS:

- 2 lb. chicken thighs
- ½ mug balsamic vinegar
- 6 cloves garlic, minced
- 2 teaspoon oregano
- 2 teaspoon Italian parsley dash black pepper
- 10 oz. baby spinach

INSTRUCTIONS:

1. Put the chicken in the cooking pan. Stir all the ingredients other than the spinach & throw it in the cooking pan. Cook for 6-7 hrs on low.

2. Put in the spinach 20 Mins prior to completion of cooking.

39. Pan Sweet & Spicy Chicken Legs

Prep Time: 10 Mins | Cooking Time: 30 Mins |
Serve: 2

INGREDIENTS:

- 2-3 lbs. chicken legs Olive oil
- ½ onion, chopped
- 5-6 cloves garlic, smashed
- 1 tablespoon cumin
- 1 tablespoon cinnamon
- 1 teaspoon coriander
- 1 teaspoon paprika
- 3-4 tablespoon white wine

INSTRUCTIONS:

1. Put olive oil in a pan & brown the chicken legs on it.
2. Put the chicken in the pan & put in the garlic, spreading it on the chicken.
3. Sauté the onions in the pan & put the spices to it & stir for some time.

4. Put in the onion batter to the chicken. Pour the white wine into the pan, deglaze it & then pour it into the cooking pan.
5. Cook the chicken for 3-4 hrs on high.

40. Pan Hot Chicken Wings

Prep Time: 15 Mins | Cooking Time: 25 Mins |
Serve: 3

INGREDIENTS:

- 3 lbs. chicken wings
- ½ mug coconut oil, melted
- ½ mug Red Hot Sauce
- ¼ mug apple cider vinegar
- ½ teaspoon paprika
- ¼ teaspoon black pepper

INSTRUCTIONS:

1. Set the oven to broil for around 10 mins.
2. Put the chicken in a safe broil pan & broil on each side for around 5 mins.
3. Combine the coconut oil, hot sauce, apple cider vinegar, paprika & black pepper in a casserole & put in a microwave for 2 mins & stir well.
4. Grease the pan with coconut oil & put in the chicken wings to it.
5. Pour the sauce over the chicken & toss the wings.
6. Cook the chicken for 2 hrs on high.

41. Pan Salsa Chicken

Prep Time: 15 Mins | Cooking Time: 20 Mins |
Serve: 2

INGREDIENTS:

- 2 mugs salsa
- 4 chicken breasts, bones removed
- 1 tablespoon chili powder
- 1 onion, chopped

INSTRUCTIONS:

1. Stir all the ingredients in a cooking pan.
2. Cook for around 8 hrs on low.

42. Pan Picante Chicken

Prep Time: 20 Mins | Cooking Time: 25 Mins |
Serve: 2

INGREDIENTS:

- Refrigerated butter-flavored cooking spray
- 1 3 ½-lb. frying chicken, cut into 10 pieces, skin removed & discarded
- 1 medium onion, diced
- 1 medium green bell pepper, seeded & diced
- 2 large cloves garlic, minced
- 3 sprigs fresh thyme or ½ teaspoon
- crushed dried thyme
- 2 to 2 ½ teaspoons curry powder
- 1 14 ½-oz. can no-salt-added diced tomatoes
- 1 teaspoon celery flakes
- 1 packet sugar substitute that will retain sweetness during long cooking
- 2 teaspoons white wine vinegar 2 Tablespoons currants

INSTRUCTIONS:

1. Take a frying pan & use spray oil to coat it.
2. Put the chicken in & fry for 5mins each side.

3. In the 4-quart cooking pan, put in the onion, bell pepper, & garlic.
4. Put the golden chicken on top, with the thyme sprigs.
5. Use a casserole & blend together the curry powder, tomatoes, celery flakes, sugar sub & wine vinegar.
6. Tip this stir over the chicken, & put in the currants, do not stir.
7. Put the lid on & cook for 7hrs on low or 3hrs on high. Finish with rice.

43. Pan d Cajun Chicken

Prep Time: 15 Mins | Cooking Time: 30 Mins |
Serve: 2

INGREDIENTS:

- 1 1/2lb To 2lb chicken—
- meaty (breasts, thighs,
- drumstick) Nonstick spray coating
- 2 tbsp. Nonfat milk
- 2 tbsp. Onion powder
- ½ Dried thyme—crushed ¼ teaspoon Garlic salt
- 1/8 teaspoon To ¼ teaspoon ground white pepper
- 1/8 teaspoon To ¼ teaspoon ground black pepper

INSTRUCTIONS:

1. Preheat the oven to 375 F
2. Take the chicken & clean, wash under the tap, & take the skin off.
3. Grease a 13"×9"×2" baking tray with spray oil.
4. Put the chicken in, & smear with milk.
5. Stir together the onion powder, thyme, garlic salt, red, white & black pepper.
6. Dust this over the chicken.

7. Put in the oven & cook for 50mins, or when the chicken is cooked through.

44. Pan Pepperoni Chicken

Prep Time: 10 Mins | Cooking Time: 20 Mins |
Serve: 2

INGREDIENTS:

- 3 ½-4 lbs. meaty chicken pieces (breast halves, thighs, & drumsticks), skinned
- 1/8 teaspoon salt
- 1/8 teaspoon black pepper
- 2 oz. sliced turkey pepperoni
- ¼ mug sliced pitted ripe olives
- ½ mug reduced-sodium chicken broth
- 1 Tablespoon tomato paste
- 1 teaspoon dried Italian seasoning, crushed ½ mug shredded part-skim mozzarella cheese (2 oz.)

INSTRUCTIONS:

1. Season the chicken, & put it into a 4-quart cooking pan.
2. Slice the pepperoni into 2, & put in the cooker with the olives. Take a casserole, & stir together the broth, tomato paste, & Italian seasoning.

3. Pour into the cooker, put the lid on, & cook on low for 7hrs or high for 3 1/2hrs.
4. When done, take out the chicken, olives, & pepperoni, put it on the serving platter.
5. Dust the chicken with cheese, & cover, let it rest for 5mins, then enjoy.

45. Pan Lemon Chicken with Stuffing

Prep Time: 15 Mins | Cooking Time: 25 Mins | Serve: 3

INGREDIENTS:

- 2 tablespoons finely shredded lemon peel
- 1 Tablespoon ground sage
- ½ teaspoon seasoned salt
- ½ teaspoon freshly ground black pepper
- 8 small chicken legs (drumstick & thigh), skinned (about 5 lbs.)
- ¼ mug olive oil
- 4 mugs quartered or sliced fresh cremini, shiitake, and/or button mushrooms
- 2 cloves garlic, thinly sliced
- 8 mugs sourdough baguette cut into 1-inch pieces (12 to 14 oz.)
- 1 mug coarsely shredded carrot
- 1 mug reduced-sodium chicken broth
- ¼ mug chopped walnuts, toasted
- ¼ mug snipped flat-leaf Italian parsley

INSTRUCTIONS:

1. Use the spray oil, & grease the inner pot of a 6-quart cooker.

2. Keep 1 teaspoon of lemon peel, put in the rest to a casserole along with the sage & seasoning.

3. Smear ¾ of the stir onto the chicken pieces, & put in the cooker.

4. In a large frying pan, warm the oil, & fry the mushrooms & garlic for 4mins.

5. Then put in the sage mix, & blend well. In a larger casserole, put in the bread, and

6. carrots, stir & put the mushrooms in. Stir again, along with the broth, put the stir over the chicken.

7. Put the lid on & switch to high, cook for 4hrs.

8. Once cooked, remove the chicken & stuffing from the cooker to a platter. You do not need the stock in the cooker.

9. Blend the remaining lemon peel with walnuts & parsley. Put over the chicken.

46. Pan-Broiled Steak

Prep Time: 15 Mins | Cooking Time: 25 Mins |
Serve: 2

INGREDIENTS:

- 1 ½ pound (680 g) steak, 1-inch (2.5 cm) thick—
  We like rib eye, but T-bone, sirloin, or strip will
  all do.
- 1 tbsp. bacon grease (15 g) or olive oil (15 ml)

DIRECTIONS:

1. Place your big, heavy pan—cast iron is best—on
   highest heat & let it get good & hot. In the
   meantime, you can season your steak if you like.
   We like the Montreal Steak Seasoning that's
   currently popular, or you could use Southwestern
   Steak Rub or the Cocoa-Chili Rub on anything
   you like.

2. Or instead, you could top it when done with the
   Bacon-Butter, or butter & blue cheese, or
   sautéed onions & mushrooms, or go for classic
   simplicity & just Salt & pepper it.

3. When the pan's hot, add the bacon grease or oil
   & slosh it around & then throw in your steak. Set
   a timer for 5 to 6 mins—your timing will depend

on your taste & how hot your burner gets, but on my stove, 5 mins per side with a 1-inch (2.5 cm) thick steak comes out medium-rare. When it's done, flip the steak & set the timer again. When time is up, devour immediately!

47. Rib Eye Steak with Wine Sauce

Prep Time: 15 Mins | Cooking Time: 25 Mins |
Serve: 2

INGREDIENTS:

- 1 tbsp. (15 ml) olive oil
- 1 ½ pound (680 g) beef rib eye
- 2 shallots
- ½ cup (120 ml) dry red wine
- ½ cup (120 ml) beef stock, or ½ cup (120 ml) water & ½ teaspoon beef bouillon concentrate 1 tbsp. (15 ml) balsamic vinegar
- 1 teaspoon brown mustard, or Dijon
- 1 tbsp. (4 g) dried thyme
- 3 tbsps. (42 g) butter
- salt & pepper to taste

DIRECTIONS:

1. Cook your steak as described in Pan Broiled Steak.
2. In the meantime, assemble everything for your wine sauce—chop your shallots & measure the wine, beef stock, vinegar, mustard, & thyme

together in a measuring cup with a pouring lip. Whisk them up.

3. When it's done, flip the steak & set the timer again.

4. When your steak is done, place it on a platter. Pour the wine batter into the pan & stir it around, scraping up the nice brown bits, & let it boil hard.

5. Continue boiling your sauce until it's reduced by at least half. Melt in the butter, Salt & pepper, & serve with your steak.

48. Salmon With Caper Sauce

Prep Time: 15 Mins | Cooking Time: 25 Mins | Serve: 2

INGREDIENTS:

- 3 salmon fillets
- Salt and black pepper to the taste
- 1 Tbsp. olive oil
- 1 Tbsp. Italian seasoning
- 2 Tbsps. capers
- 3 Tbsps. lemon juice
- 4 garlic cloves, minced
- 2 Tbsps. ghee

INSTRUCTIONS:

1. Warm up a pot with the olive oil on medium to high heat, put in fish fillets skin side up, season them with salt, pepper, and Italian seasoning, cook for 2 mins, flip and cook for 2 more mins, take off heat, con pot and leave aside for 15 mins.

2. Transfer fish to a plate and leave them aside.

3. Warm up the same pot on medium to high heat, put in capers, lemon juice, and garlic, stir and cook for 2 mins.
4. Take the pot off the heat, put in ghee, and stir very well.
5. Return fish to the pot and toss to coat with the sauce.
6. Divide between plates and serve. Enjoy!

49. Simple Grilled Oysters

Prep Time: 15 Mins | Cooking Time: 25 Mins |
Serve: 2

INGREDIENTS:

- 6 big oysters, shucked
- 3 garlic cloves, minced
- 1 lemon cut in wedges
- 1 Tbsp. parsley
- A pinch of sweet paprika
- 2 Tbsps. melted ghee

INSTRUCTIONS:

1. Top each oyster with melted ghee, parsley, paprika, and ghee.
2. Place them on the preheated grill on medium to high heat and cook for 8 mins.
3. Serve them with lemon wedges on the side.
4. Enjoy!

50. Baked Halibut

Prep Time: 15 Mins | Cooking Time: 25 Mins | Serve: 2

INGREDIENTS:

- ½ cup parmesan, grated
- ¼ cup ghee
- ¼ cup mayonnaise
- 2 Tbsps. green onions
- 6 garlic cloves, minced
- A dash of Tabasco sauce
- 4 halibut fillets
- Salt and black pepper to the taste
- Juice of ½ lemon

INSTRUCTIONS:

1. Season halibut with salt, pepper, and some of the lemon juice, place in a baking dish, and cook in the oven at 450 F for 6 mins.
2. Meanwhile, Warm up a pot with the ghee on medium to high heat, put in parmesan, mayo, green onions, Tabasco sauce, garlic, and the rest of the lemon juice, and stir well.

3. Take fish out of the oven, drizzle parmesan sauce all on, turn oven to broil, and broil your fish for 3 mins.
4. Divide between plates and serve.

51. Pan Chicken Dumplings

Prep Time: 20 Mins | Cooking Time: 25 Mins |
Serve: 2

INGREDIENTS:

- 1 (3 lb.) chicken
- Salt & pepper
- 2 cloves garlic, minced
- ¼ teaspoon powdered marjoram
- ¼ teaspoon powdered thyme
- 1 bay leaf
- ½ mug dry white wine (optional)
- 1 mug dairy sour cream
- 1 mug packaged biscuit mix
- 1 Tablespoon chopped parsley
- 6 Tablespoons milk
- 10 small white onions

INSTRUCTIONS:

1. Season the chicken with salt and
2. pepper.
3. Leave for a few mins & put in the cooking pan.

4. Imbed the cloves gently into one onion & put all the onions with the meat. Stir in the garlic, thyme, marjoram, bay leaf & wine.

5. Put lid & cook for 5 hrs on low & once cooked take out the cloves & the bay leaf.

6. Put in the sour cream & stir well. Stir the parsley, biscuit, stir, and the milk together & increase to High. Drop the dumplings gently from about 1 teaspoon away from the corner of the pot. Leave covered for another 30 mins.

52. Homemade Pan Chicken 'n' Dumplings

Prep Time: 20 Mins | Cooking Time: 20 Mins |
Serve: 3

INGREDIENTS:

- 2 mugs cooked chicken
- 1 can (10 ¾ oz.) condensed cream of mushroom soup, undiluted
- 1 can (10 ¾ oz.) condensed cream of chicken soup, undiluted
- 2 soup cans water
- 4 teaspoon all-purpose flour
- 2 teaspoon chicken bouillon granules
- ½ teaspoon black pepper
- 1 can refrigerated buttermilk biscuits (8 biscuits)

INSTRUCTIONS:

1. Put all the ingredients, excluding the buttermilk biscuits, in a cooking pan.
2. Slice the biscuits into 4 & toss them into the cooking pan.
3. Cover with lid & allow to cook for 6 hrs on low.

53. Pan Western Dump Chicken

Prep Time: 15 Mins | Cooking Time: 25 Mins |
Serve: 2

INGREDIENTS:

- 2 (15 ¼ oz.) cans kernel corn, drained
- 1 (15 oz.) can black beans, rinsed & drained
- 1 (16 oz.) jar chunky salsa, divided
- 6 boneless skinless chicken breast halves
- 1 mug (4 oz.) shredded Cheddar cheese

INSTRUCTIONS:

1. Put the black beans, corn & ½ the quantity of the salsa in a cooking pan.
2. Top up with chicken & put in the balance salsa over the ingredients. Cook for 8 hrs on low until the meat
3. is tender.
4. Sprinkle with shredded cheese & leave for 5 mins.

54. Crock Pit Chicken Broccoli

Prep Time: 15 Mins | Cooking Time: 25 Mins |
Serve: 2

INGREDIENTS:

- 4 to 6 boneless skinless chicken breasts
- 1 small box Stove Top Stuffing for chicken
- 1 (10 oz.) package frozen chopped broccoli, thawed
- 1 can broccoli with cheese soup
- ½ mug chicken broth
- Lightly butter a 3 ½-quart pan & put the chicken on the bottom

INSTRUCTIONS:

1. Put the ingredients & the chicken in the cooking pan.
2. Cover with lid & cook for 6-7 hrs on low.

55. Pan Cinnamon Chicken

***Prep Time: 20 Mins | Cooking Time: 30 Mins |
Serve: 2***

INGREDIENTS:

- 2 lb. chicken breasts
- 2 Bell Peppers sliced
- 1 Onion diced
- 2 teaspoon Paprika
- 4 cloves garlic minced
- 2 teaspoon cinnamon
- 1 Mug Chicken broth
- ¼ teaspoon Nutmeg

INSTRUCTIONS:

1. Put all ingredients into a pan & cook for 4 hrs on high or 6 hrs on low.

56. Pan Chicken Pad Thai

Prep Time: 15 Mins | Cooking Time: 25 Mins |
Serve: 3

INGREDIENTS:

- 2 to 3 lbs. of chicken breasts
- 2 medium zucchini
- 1 large carrot
- 1 handful of bean sprouts
- 1 small bunch of green onions (for sauce & garnish)
- 1 mug of coconut milk
- 1 mug of chicken stock
- 2 heaping Tablespoons of Sun Butter
- 1 tablespoon of Coconut Aminos
- 2 teaspoons of Paleo friendly Red boat Fish Sauce.
- 2 teaspoon of powdered ginger
- 2 cloves of garlic, smashed and
- minced
- 1 teaspoon of cayenne pepper
- 1 teaspoon of red pepper flakes
- Salt & pepper for seasoning the chicken

- Chopped cashews for garnish Chopped cilantro for garnish

INSTRUCTIONS:

1. Season the chicken with cayenne pepper, ginger powder, salt & pepper. Put the coconut milk & the chicken stock in the pan & stir well. Put in the coconut aminos, Sun Butter, fish sauce, garlic, ginger, two chopped green onions, cayenne & red pepper & stir until the sun butter completely

2. dissolves.

3. Put the chicken breasts in the liquid. Slice the zucchini spirally & shred the carrot.

4. Combine the zucchini, carrots & bean sprouts & put them on top of the meat. Cook on low for 3 ½ to 4 hrs. Remove the veggies first & set them aside in the serving dish. Remove the chicken & put on the veggies.

5. Sprinkle some of the broth from the pan on top & garnish with chopped green onions, cashews & cilantro.

57. Pan Red Pepper Pulled Chicken

***Prep Time: 20 Mins | Cooking Time: 25 Mins |
Serve: 2***

INGREDIENTS:

- 2.5 to 3 lbs. of boneless & skinless chicken breasts
- 2 lbs. of red bell peppers, seeded & roasted in olive oil
- 12 cloves of garlic
- 1 mug of tomato sauce ½ teaspoon oregano
- ½ teaspoon basil
- ½ teaspoon thyme
- 1 mug of water
- 1 medium white onion, chopped very fine

INSTRUCTIONS:

1. Put the onion, tomato sauce & water into the pan & stir.
2. Put in the oregano, basil & thyme & mix.
3. Use a fork & hole the chicken & stuff some of the garlic cloves.

4. Put the chicken breasts in the pan so that it is submerged in the gravy. Put the roasted red peppers & roast the remaining garlic cloves & put over the chicken.
5. Cook for 4-5 hrs on low.
6. Remove the chicken from the pan & shred.
7. Remove the roasted peppers & put them into a blender & pulse blend until you get a
8. chunky texture.
9. Put the shredded chicken, topped with the roasted peppers & a drizzle of the broth left in the pan in the serving casserole.

58. Pan Buffalo Chicken & Eggplant Lasagna

Prep Time: 15 Mins | Cooking Time: 20 Mins |
Serve: 2

INGREDIENTS:

- 2 lbs. of boneless chicken breasts
- 1 large purple eggplant, sliced medium thin
- 1 mug of Frank's Red Hot Sauce
- 1 medium white onion, sliced thin
- 2 to 4 mugs of fresh baby spinach
- 1 /2 to 1 mug of crumbled bleu cheese
- 4 garlic cloves, minced
- Salt, pepper, & parsley to season the chicken

INSTRUCTIONS:

1. Slice the eggplant & put in a casserole of water to soak.
2. Chop the chicken into chunks & lb. them thin.
3. Season the chicken with salt, pepper & parsley.
4. Combine the hot sauce, minced garlic, onion slices & chicken in a casserole & toss.
5. Strain the eggplant & dry with kitchen towels.

6. Layer the pan with some sauce, then the eggplant slices & then the chicken & spinach & then repeat the layering.
7. Cook for 5 hrs on low or 3 hrs on high.

59. Pan Cheesy Dump Chicken Nachos

Prep Time: 15 Mins | Cooking Time: 30 Mins |
Serve: 2

INGREDIENTS:

- 1 small bag of tortilla chips
- 4 to 6 chicken breasts
- 1 mug Picante sauce
- 2 mugs Monterey Jack cheese, grated
- ½ mug sour cream ½ mug guacamole

INSTRUCTIONS:

1. Put tortilla chips in a cooking pan. Lay the chicken on the layer of the tortilla chips.

2. Pour the sauce over the ingredients—Cook for about 8 hrs on low. Toss in the grated cheese & leave until the cheese becomes melted.

3. Transfer from the pan & serve with guacamole, sour cream & tortilla chips.

60. Pan Spicy Dump Chicken

Prep Time: 20 Mins | Cooking Time: 25 Mins |
Serve: 3

INGREDIENTS:

- 1 value-pack chicken
- 1 Tablespoon olive oil
- 1 Tablespoon lime juice
- 2 Tablespoon orange juice
- 2 Tablespoon lemon juice
- 2 Tablespoon chili powder
- 2 Tablespoon paprika
- 1 teaspoon cayenne
- ¼ teaspoon pepper
- ¼ teaspoon salt

INSTRUCTIONS:

1. Put the chicken in the cooking pan. Stir the rest of the ingredients & put them on to the chicken.
2. Leave for about 6 hrs on low until the meat is tender.
3. Serve with rice & veggies.

61. Pan General Tsao's Dump Chicken

Prep Time: 15 Mins | Cooking Time: 25 Mins |
Serve: 2

INGREDIENTS:

- 4 boneless skinless chicken breasts
- ½ mug water
- 3 Tablespoon hoisin sauce
- 2 Tablespoon soy sauce
- ½ mug brown sugar
- 3 Tablespoon ketchup
- ¼ teaspoon dry ginger
- ½ teaspoon crushed red pepper (more or less to liking)
- 1 Tablespoon cornstarch

INSTRUCTIONS:

1. Stir the sugar, sauces, ketchup, ginger & red pepper in a casserole.
2. Spray the pan using a cooking
3. spray & put the chicken breasts in the cooking pan.

4. Pour the batter over the chicken breasts & cook on low for about 6 hrs.

5. Transfer the chicken onto a board & slice into chunks.

6. Stir in the cornstarch to the sauce & whisk well.

7. Put the chicken breasts into the pan & leave for another 20 Mins to heat through.

8. Serve with rice & sprinkle with sesame seeds if required.

62. Pan Lemon Dump Chicken

Prep Time: 20 Mins | Cooking Time: 20 Mins |
Serve: 3

INGREDIENTS:

- 4 boneless skinless chicken breast halves (or cut into tenders) 1/8 mug extra virgin olive oil
- ½ Tablespoon dill seasoning juice from ½ of a lemon
- 1-2 Teaspoon minced garlic (depending on how garlic-y you want the taste)

INSTRUCTIONS:

1. Put the ingredients into the pan & cook on low for about 6 hrs until the meat is tender.

63. Pan BBQ Pulled Chicken

Prep Time: 20 Mins | Cooking Time: 20 Mins |
Serve: 3

INGREDIENTS:

- 6 Boneless, Skinless Chicken Thighs
- 1/3 Mug Salted Butter ¼ Mug Erythritol
- ¼ Mug Red Wine Vinegar ¼ Mug Chicken Stock
- ¼ Mug Organic Tomato Paste 2 Tablespoon Yellow Mustard
- 2 Tablespoon Spicy Brown Mustard
- 1 Tablespoon Liquid Smoke
- 1 Tablespoon Soy Sauce
- 2 teaspoon Chili Powder
- 1 teaspoon Cumin
- 1 teaspoon Cayenne Pepper
- 1 teaspoon Red Boat Fish Sauce

INSTRUCTIONS:

1. In a casserole, put together all ingredients except for butter & chicken thighs.

2. Put frozen (or fresh) chicken thighs in a pan & pour sauce over them. If you AREN'T going to be home, turn your pan to low, put in butter & leave for 7-10 hrs.

3. If you ARE going to be home, turn your pan to low for 2 hrs & put in the butter. Then turn to high, & cook for an additional 3 hrs.

4. Once your chicken has cooked down, shred the chicken with 2 forks. Put in sauce & stir well.

5. Turn pan to high & cook for additional 45 mins.

64. VEGETABLE SOUP FOR THE HEART

Prep Time: 20 Mins | Cooking Time: 20 Mins |
Serve: 3

INGREDIENTS:

- You can control the cooking or the spray
- One medium onion, see two cloves, thinly sliced
- Two thick, trimmed and thin sticks
- Two medium slices or two peppers, cut into two pieces / 1 in pieces 400 g / 14 ounces canned tomatoes
- One bucket of stock vegetables
- One tablespoon of mixed herbs
- 400 g / 14 ounces of tin butter are seasoned and rinsed
- One head of thin plants (approximately 125 g / 4½ ounces), cut and veiled said and ground freshly ground pepper

INSTRUCTIONS:

1. Spray a large amount of nonstick with oil and see the rest, sauce, sauce, and carrots or peppers gently for 10 minutes; keep stirring until they soften.

2. Add 750 ml / 26 ounces at a time and the other chopped. Crumble after the fat is gone and mix in the dry flavors.

3. Bring the bile, then recover the form of simmering and wait 20 minutes. Season the soup with salt and soda and add the excellent plums and fillings.

4. Return to a tasty sauce and cook for another 3-4 minutes or until the vegetables soften. I thought about trying and serving in many specialties.

65. LAMB AND FLAGELLET LAMB BEANS

Prep Time: 20 Mins | Cooking Time: 20 Mins |
Serve: 3

INGREDIENTS:

- One teaspoon of oil
- 350 g / 12 oz and to the left, according
- 16 crispy onions
- One garlic left, crushed
- 600 ml / 20 ml large broth (produced with a sufficient quantity of food)
- 200 g can choose
- One because you are Garni
- 2 x 400 g can be dried beans, seasoned and rinsed
- 320 g / 11 green ounces
- 250 g / 9 ounces really should
- Fresh and abundant pepper black

INSTRUCTIONS:

1. He took the oil in an instant spell or, even later, left the liquor and fried for 3-4 minutes until it was all over.

2. Remove the lamb from the pan and set it aside. Add the first and most often to the pan and fry for 4-5 minutes, or until the onions begin to brown.
3. Return all the pieces to the pan. Add the stock, tomatoes, bouquet garni, and beans.
4. Carry the ball, stir, then before and some time for 1 hour, or until the lamb is only tender.
5. Hurry up, boil a pot of water and blanch the beans. Put in a bowl with ice water.
6. Add the crispy tomatoes to the sauce and season with freshly ground white pepper.
7. Continue shooting for 10 minutes. Divide the stew into four dishes; also, set the beans aside and leave them.
8. Recipe tips could be done the night before and then overheated.

66. CHERRY PACK AND CHERRY FISH

Prep Time: 20 Mins | Cooking Time: 20 Mins | Serve: 3

INGREDIENTS:

- 125 g / 4½ oz of steak, little or little steak
- Two tablespoons of juice
- One tablespoon first
- One garlic, freshly chopped
- One grated studied and chopped
- ¼ teaspoon of sugar
- Two tablespoons of natural yogurt
- 80 g / 3 minutes must think to serve

INSTRUCTIONS:

1. Remove the oven at 200° C / 180° Fas / Gays 6. Taste the flavor in a way not too long and stick with the lemon juice.
2. Cover & leave in the refrigerator for 15-20 min. Put the garlic, the garlic, and the red pepper in one good dose of meat and process until the mixture strengthened.

3. Add some sugar, yogurt, and apply the fusion process briefly. Put the meat in a good dose of the fetus. Make part of both sides with the paste.
4. Collect the tissue without tightening and give the back to seal it. Keep it in the refrigerator for 1 hour.
5. Let stand on a baking sheet and cook for about 15 minutes, or until the dish has prepared— Swabians with scabies.

Conclusion

Thank you again for purchasing this book!

I hope this book was able to help you discover some amazing Pan Recipes. The next step is to get cooking!!!

CPSIA information can be obtained
at www.ICGtesting.com
Printed in the USA
BVHW092333240621
610373BV00004B/908